P9-AFE-597

These quotations were gathered lovingly but unscientifically over several years and/or contributed by many friends or acquaintances. Some arrived, and survived in our files, on scraps of paper and may therefore be imperfectly worded or attributed. To the authors, contributors and original sources, our thanks, and where appropriate, our apologies. —The Editors

CREDITS

Compiled by Dan Zadra
Designed by Steve Potter

ISBN: 978-1-932319-69-9

©2008 Compendium, Incorporated. All rights reserved. No part of this publication may be reproduced or transmitted in any form or by any means, electronic or mechanical, including photocopy, recording, or any storage and retrieval system now known or to be invented without written permission from the publisher. Contact: Compendium, Inc., 600 North 36th Street, Suite 400, Seattle, WA 98103. Hope, The Good Life, Celebrating the Joy of Living Fully, Compendium, live inspired and the format, design, layout and coloring used in this book are trademarks and/or trade dress of Compendium, Incorporated. This book may be ordered directly from the publisher, but please try your local bookstore first. Call us at 800-91-IDEAS or come see our full line of inspiring products at www.live-inspired.com. 1st Printing. 10K 04 08

Printed in China

There will come a time when

you believe everything is finished.

That will be the beginning.

LOUIS L'AMOUR

I have walked the road ahead and come back to tell all cancer patients that there is hope — and where there is hope, all things are possible.

VICKIE GIRARD,
"THERE'S NO PLACE LIKE HOPE"

WE ARE WINNING THE WAR

ON CANCER, THAT'S FOR SURE.

ALMOST EVERY WEEK BRINGS

NEWS OF ANOTHER PROMISING

INSIGHT OR ADVANCEMENT.

CONNIE PAYTON,
"STRONGER THAN CANCER"

Through the

centuries,

we faced

down death

by daring

to hope.

MAYA ANGELOU

You gain strength, courage and confidence by every experience in which you really stop to look fear in the face. You must do the thing you think you cannot do.

ELEANOR ROOSEVELT

KNOWLEDGE
IS THE ANTIDOTE TO FEAR.

RALPH WALDO EMERSON

NOTHING IN LIFE IS TO BE FEARED,
IT IS ONLY TO BE
UNDERSTOOD.
NOW IS THE TIME
TO UNDERSTAND MORE,
SO THAT WE CAN
FEAR LESS.

MARIE CURIE

We have the ability
to face adversity —
to come from behind
and win with grace.

AMBER BROOKMAN

Believe that problems do have answers, that they can be overcome, and that we can solve them.

NORMAN VINCENT PEALE

As for courage and will—

we cannot measure

how much of each lies within us,

we can only trust that

it will be sufficient

to carry us through trials

which may lie ahead.

ANDRE NORTON

Have faith. Your creator will never give you a problem or an opportunity without at the same time providing every-thing you need to handle it.

DAN ZADRA

IF CHILDREN HAVE THE ABILITY
TO IGNORE ALL ODDS AND
PERCENTAGES, THEN MAYBE
WE CAN ALL LEARN FROM
THEM. WHEN YOU THINK ABOUT
IT, WHAT OTHER CHOICE IS
THERE BUT TO HOPE. WE HAVE
TWO OPTIONS, MEDICALLY
AND EMOTIONALLY: GIVE
UP, OR FIGHT LIKE HELL.

LANCE ARMSTRONG

I have heard there are troubles

of more than one kind.

Some come from ahead and

some come from behind.

But I've brought a big bat.

I'm all ready you see.

Now my troubles are going

to have troubles with me!

DR. SEUSS

THERE IS NO SUCH THING
AS NO CHANCE.

HENRY FORD

No matter what the statistics say there is always a way.

BERNIE SIEGEL

The biggest
obstacle
to overcoming
the odds
is never
challenging them.

ROB GILBERT

When everything you know
says you can't.

When everything within you
says you can't.

Dig deep within yourself, find it,
and you can.

MARK   ELLIOTT   SACKS

HARDSHIP
OFTEN PREPARES
AN ORDINARY PERSON FOR AN
EXTRAORDINARY DESTINY.

C.S. LEWIS

The illness caused all the greatness in her to rise to the surface.

MARY STEENBURGEN

We need to teach our children that not all heroes are honored in the big parades. There are everyday people all across the country —

doctors, nurses and patients — who are quietly battling cancer and whose courage would easily eclipse the caped crusaders'.

TERRI ATKINSON

A HERO IS JUST

AN ORDINARY

INDIVIDUAL

WHO FINDS THE

STRENGTH TO

PERSEVERE

IN SPITE OF

OVERWHELMING

OBSTACLES.

CHRISTOPHER REEVE

I am here. Let's heal together.

UNKNOWN

People
come together
because they
need each other
and they need
to hear
victories
about each other.

BILL MILLIKEN

FRIENDS ARE GOD'S WAY
OF TAKING CARE OF US.

UNKNOWN

I believe in angels

The kind that heaven sends

I'm surrounded by angels

But I call them my best friends.

UNKNOWN

DRAW STRENGTH
FROM EACH OTHER.

JAMES A. RENIER

Cancer begins with a "C,"
but the dictionary has a lot
of "C" words. They include
Compassion, Confidence,
Courage and Cuddles.

LINDA SCOTT

We need
heart-to-heart
resuscitation.

RAM DASS

If someone listens,

or stretches out a hand,

or whispers a kind

word of encouragement,

or attempts to understand,

extraordinary things

begin to happen.

LORETTA GIRZARTIS

ENCOURAGEMENT IS OXYGEN FOR THE SOUL.

A N O N Y M O U S

Friends feed each other's spirits and dreams and hopes; they feed each other with the things a soul needs to live.

GLEN HARRINGTON-HALL

There is no difficulty
that enough love
will not conquer; no
disease that enough
love will not heal; no
door that enough
love will not open.

EMMET FOX

IN TIMES OF DARKNESS
LOVE SEES,

IN TIMES OF SILENCE
LOVE HEARS,

IN TIMES OF DOUBT
LOVE HOPES,

IN TIMES OF SORROW
LOVE HEALS…

UNKNOWN

WARNING:

LAUGHTER MAY BE

HAZARDOUS TO

YOUR ILLNESS.

NURSES FOR LAUGHTER

LAUGHTER

AND CRYING ARE

TWO OF THE BEST

HEALERS WE HAVE.

PETER McWILLIAMS

There are no hopeless situations; there are only people who have grown hopeless about them.

CLARE BOOTH LUCE

HOPE NEVER ABANDONS YOU,
YOU ABANDON IT.

GEORGE WEINBERG

God's delays are not God's denials.

REVEREND JAMES CLEVELAND

Be patient. It is astonishing how

short a time it can take for very

wonderful things to happen.

FRANCES H. BURNETT

We may
encounter
many defeats,
but we
must not be
defeated.

MAYA ANGELOU

YOU DO WHAT YOU
CAN FOR AS LONG
AS YOU CAN, AND
WHEN YOU FINALLY
CAN'T, YOU DO THE
NEXT BEST THING.
YOU BACK UP, BUT
YOU DON'T GIVE UP.

CHUCK YEAGER

In the depth of winter,

I finally learned

that within me lies

an invincible summer.

ALBERT CAMUS

GOALS
ARE LIKE STARS—
THEY ARE ALWAYS THERE.
ADVERSITY
IS LIKE A CLOUD—
IT MOVES ON.
KEEP YOUR EYES ON THE STARS.

DON WARD

A negative attitude

is the only true handicap.

SCOTT HAMILTON, CANCER SURVIVOR

Attitudes are

more important than facts.

DR. KARL A. MENNINGER

I WILL SAY THIS ABOUT BEING AN OPTIMIST — EVEN WHEN THINGS DON'T TURN OUT WELL, YOU ARE CERTAIN THEY WILL GET BETTER.

FRANK HUGHES

Perpetual optimism is a force multiplier.

COLIN POWELL

Every life has
its dark and
joyful hours.
Happiness
comes from
choosing
which to
remember.

UNKNOWN

Please, Lord,

teach us to

laugh again;

but God, don't

ever let us forget

that we cried.

BILL WILSON

Have faith.
God's care will carry
you...so you can
carry others.

DR. ROBERT H. SCHULLER

You do build in darkness if you have faith. But one day the light returns and you discover that you have become a fortress which is impregnable to certain kinds of trouble; you may even find yourself needed and sought by others as a beacon in their dark.

OLGA ROSMANITH

ALTHOUGH THE WORLD IS FULL OF SUFFERING, IT'S ALSO FULL OF THE OVERCOMING OF IT.

HELEN KELLER

A SCAR IS A

REMINDER

OF SOMETHING

BAD THAT HAS

HAPPENED;

BUT A SCAR IS ALSO

A SIGN THAT

HEALING

HAS TAKEN PLACE.

UNKNOWN

This entire nation is populated by cancer survivors—everyday people who have beaten, and are beating this disease. Let their success fuel your success!

VICKIE GIRARD,
"THERE'S NO PLACE LIKE HOPE"

You are not
made for failure,
you are made
for victory.
Go forward
with joyful
confidence.

GEORGE ELIOT

MAY YOUR BURDENS BE LIGHTER
AND YOUR STAR SHINE EVEN BRIGHTER.

EARL GRAVES

AS SOON AS HEALING TAKES PLACE,
GO OUT AND HEAL SOMEBODY ELSE.

MAYA ANGELOU

the good life™

Celebrating the joy of living fully.

Also available are these spirited
companion books in The Good Life
series of great quotations:

drive
friend
heart
hero
joy
moxie
refresh
service
spirit
success
thanks
value
vision
welcome
yes!